Ghada Kharrat
Safa Jemli

Thyroid nodules

Ghada Kharrat
Safa Jemli

Thyroid nodules

echo-histological confrontation

ScienciaScripts

Cover image: www.ingimage.com

This book is a translation from the original published under ISBN 978-620-6-72278-6.

Publisher:
Sciencia Scripts
is a trademark of
Dodo Books Indian Ocean Ltd. and OmniScriptum S.R.L publishing group

120 High Road, East Finchley, London, N2 9ED, United Kingdom
Str. Armeneasca 28/1, office 1, Chisinau MD-2012, Republic of Moldova, Europe
Printed at: see last page
ISBN: 978-620-8-11283-7

TABLE OF CONTENTS

INTRODUCTION

The thyroid nodule is defined as an enlargement of the thyroid gland, which may be recognised clinically, radiologically or histologically [1] Thyroid nodules are found in 20 to 76% of the general population[2].

Most are asymptomatic[3].Despite the high prevalence of thyroid nodules, only 1.6% to 12% of cases are diagnosed. malignant [4] [5]. This significant discrepancy between the high prevalence of thyroid nodules and the low risk of malignancy encountered makes surgical exploration of all thyroid nodules inconceivable, given the risks associated with surgery and its high cost. The difficulty in managing this condition stems from the fact that only histopathological examination can confirm or rule out malignancy with certainty. Ultrasound is the reference examination of first choice for the positive diagnosis of thyroid pathology[6]. Thanks to advances in ultrasound, it allows considerable histological orientation and consequently a better therapeutic strategy, with a reduction in the number of unnecessary thyroidectomies[7]. Several ultrasound classifications have been proposed to standardise the approach to thyroid nodules. The TIRADS classification is currently the most widely used, initially proposed in 2009 by Horvath et al [8]. This classification was simplified and modified in 2017 by Russ et al [9] in order to ensure the evolutivity and continuity of the TIRADS score, with a view to simplifying the daily work of practitioners and based on the various studies carried out on thyroid nodules [9].Between 2017 and 2022, several studies investigated the reliability of the EU-TIRADS 2017 classification as a tool for predicting the malignancy of thyroid nodules and the results were not very concordant, which prompted us to carry out this work, the aim of which was to study the validity of the EU-TIRADS 2017 ultrasound classification as a means of predicting the malignancy of thyroid nodules through a radio-histological comparison.

METHODS

1. Patients and methods :

1.1.Time and place of the study :

This was a monocentric retrospective study spread over a period of 3 years from July 2017 to July 2020 including 300 patients with nodular thyroid pathology managed in the ENT and cervico-facial surgery (CCF) department of the Mohamed Taher Maâmouri University Hospital in Nabeul.

1.2.Study population :

1.2.1. Inclusion criteria :

We included the following patients in our study:

• Over the age of 16.

• Undergoing loboisthmectomy and/or total thyroidectomy for a

or several thyroid nodules during the study period

• Patients with complete files containing epidemiological and clinical data, a thyroid work-up, a cervical ultrasound scan interpreted using the EUTIRADS 2017 classification (appendix 2), and surgical and pathological anatomy reports

1.2.2. Non-inclusion criteria :

Patients were not included in our study:

• Under 16 years of age.

• Thyroid nodules not suitable for surgical treatment or operated on elsewhere than in the ENT and CCF department of the Mohamed Tahar Mâamouri University Hospital.

• Patients who have undergone cervical ultrasound elsewhere than in the medical imaging department of Mohamed Tahar Mâamouri University Hospital

- Incomplete files

2. Collection of clinical data :

Data concerning the patient's history, risk factors and physical examination (cervical examination: characteristics of the swelling, adenopathies/laryngeal endoscopy/general examination) were collated from medical observation files retrieved from the ENT archive. All these data were recorded on a pre-established data processing form (appendix 1).

3. Collection of paraclinical data :

Thyroid investigation included :

- Cervical ultrasound: This groups together the ultrasound criteria in a

score assessing malignancy: EU TIRADS 2017 score (appendix 1).

For each nodule identified, we specified :

- The size
- Echostructure and echogenicity: Hypo-, iso- or hyperechoic
- Nodule contours
- The presence or absence of intra-nodular calcifications
- Estimating the height-to-width ratio (H /l)
- The type of vascularisation
- The presence or absence of satellite adenomegaly and its characteristics

- Thyroid cytopunction.

- Thyroid scintigraphy to classify nodules as hyperfixing or hot, isofixing and hypofixing or cold.

• The usual TSH hormone assay is systematic. T4 and T3 are measured if there are signs of clinical and/or biological dysthyroidism.

• Thyrocalcitonin measurement is requested preoperatively if medullary thyroid cancer is clinically suspected.

4. Analytical study :

Data were collected using a standardised analytical form, then entered and analysed using SPSS version 21 software. We then carried out an analytical statistical study comparing the ultrasound data (EUTIRADS 2017 classification) with the final histological results, which enabled us to calculate the following parameters: sensitivity, specificity, positive predictive value and negative predictive value.For the analytical study, correlation was examined using Pearson's Chi-square correlation coefficient and, in the event of invalidity, using Fisher's two-tailed exact test. Sensitivity, specificity, PPV and NPV values were calculated using contingency tables. The significance level for P was set at 0.05.

5. Bibliographic research :

We carried out an exhaustive search of bibliographic references using the Medline and Science Directe databases. The keywords used in our bibliographic search were: thyroid nodule, ultrasound, EU-Tirads classification, Reliability, Sensitivity, Pathological anatomy. Using the system of associated references, we extended our search and other bibliographic references were collected. In this way, we have gathered over 60 articles.

6. Ethical considerations :

Given its retrospective and observational nature, this study was not subject to prior consent from the patients included. No personal conflict of interest was incompatible with the objectives of this work. All data and information from this study were entered and analysed anonymously.

RESULTS

1. Descriptive study

1.1. Epidemiological and clinical characteristics

1.1.1. Breakdown of patients by sex and age

The patients were divided into 273 (91%) females and 27 (9%) males, giving a sex ratio (M/F) of 0.1. The average age of the patients was 47.04 ± 12.58 years, with extremes of 16 and 78 years (Figure 1). The geriatric population (>65 years) accounted for 10.7% of cases.

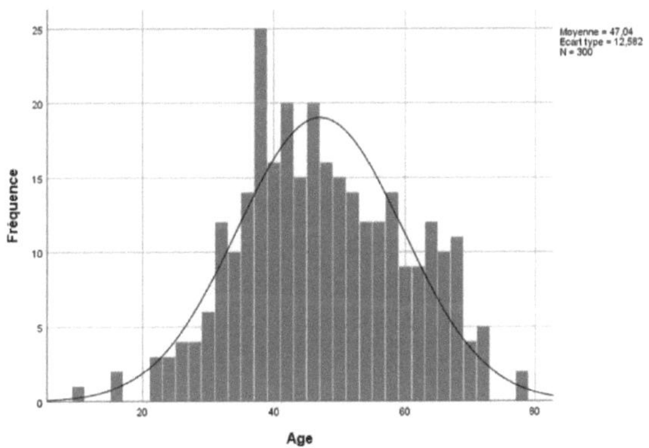

Figure 1: Breakdown of patients by age group

1.1.2. Breakdown of patients by geographical origin

The majority of patients were from north-eastern Tunisia (Figure 2).

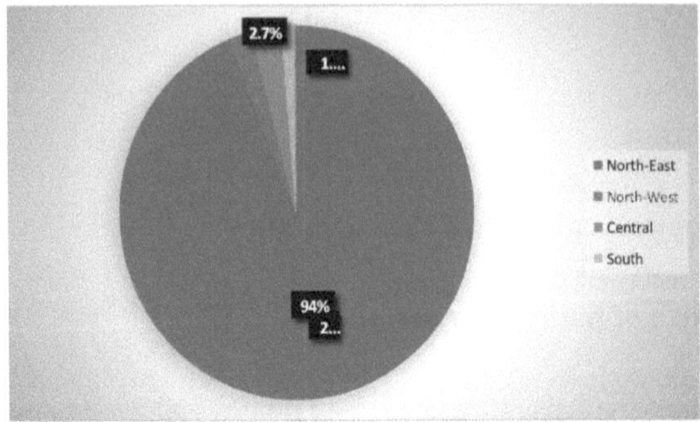

Figure 2: Breakdown of patients by geographical origin

1.1.3. Family and personal history

Forty-nine (16.33%) patients had a family history of nodular thyroid disease, malignant in 9 cases (3%). Regarding personal history, cervical irradiation was noted in 1 (0.3%) cases.

1.1.4. Deadline and reasons for consultation

The mean time to discovery of thyroid nodules was 10.55±10.84 months (range 1 month to 8 years). The most frequent reason for consultation was a finding of basicervical swelling by relatives or the patient in 80.6% of cases (Figure 3).

Resistant basedow disease in 2 patients (0.6%). % patients

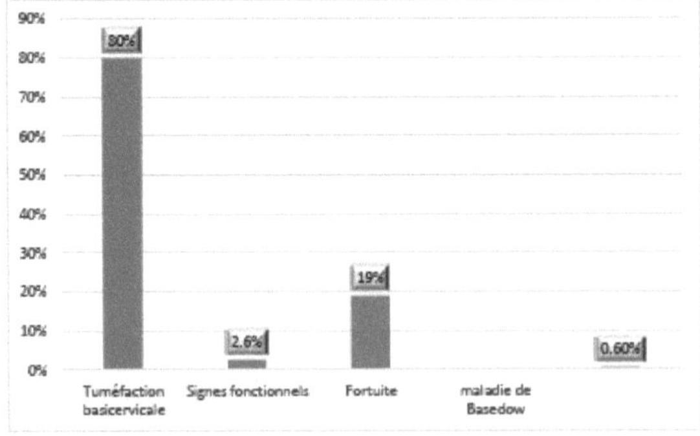

Figure 3: Distribution of patients according to the circumstances in which thyroid nodules were discovered

1.1.5. Signs functional

Only 18 patients (6%) showed signs of dysthyroidism: 12 cases of hypothyroidism and 6 cases of hyperthyroidism (including the 2 cases with a history of Graves' disease). Signs of compression were noted in 29 patients (9.7%), distributed as follows:

-dysphagia in 24 cases (8%);

-dyspnoea in 8 cases (2.7%)

-dysphonia in 2 cases (0.7%).

1.1.6. Physical examination

1.1.6.1. Examination Cervical

The mean size of the thyroid nodules was 3.59±1.55 cm (extremes 0.5 and 10 cm). Table I summarises the various characteristics of the cervical swelling found on physical examination.

Seven patients (2.3%) had cervical adenopathies, all firm and homolateral to the thyroid nodule (Table I), with a mean number per patient of 2.14±1.07 (extremes 1 and 4). The mean size of the adenopathy was 2.71±1.6 cm (extremes 1 and 5 cm).

The lymph node groups affected were distributed as follows (Figure 4):

- Group II in 3 cases;

- Group III in 4 cases;

- Group IV in 2 cases

- Group V in 2 cases.

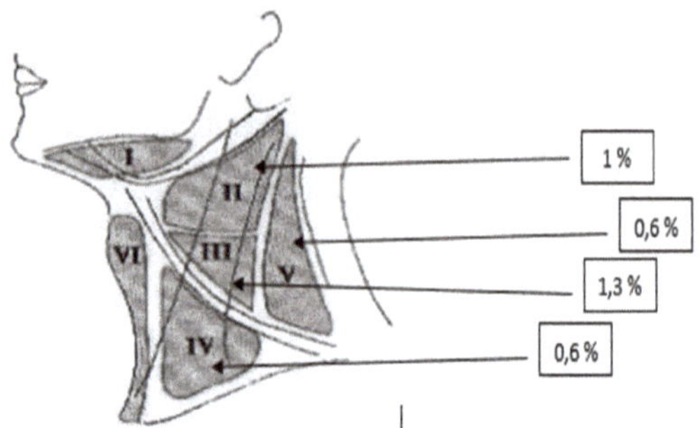

Figure 4: Lymph node grouping of adenomegaly found at cervical examination

1.1.6.2. Indirect laryngoscopy

Only one patient had vocal cord immobility homolateral to the nodule.

Table I: Clinical characteristics of thyroid nodules and cervical adenopathy

Thyroid nodules			300
Medium size	3,59 +/-155 c Farm	283	94,3
Consistency	Hard	17	5,7
Pain on palpation		0	0
Swallowing mobility		300	100
Net limits		287	95,67
Adenopathies		7	
Medium size	2.14 +/- 1.07 cm		
Headquarters	Sector II	3	1 %
	Sector III	4	1,3 %
	Sector IV	2	0,6 %
	Sector V	2	0,6 %
Laterality	Homolateral	7	100
Consistency Firm		7	100
Mobility in relation to Mobile		6	85,7
two plans Fixe		1	14,3

1.2. Data from cervical ultrasound

The majority of patients had a heterogeneous thyroid (90.3%), which was not enlarged (62%). The ultrasound data for thyroid nodules are shown in Table II.The mean size of the thyroid nodules was 28.83±12.06 mm with extremes ranging from 0.5 to 67 mm. The most frequent location was mediolobar, followed by the upper pole.On studying the echostructure (Figure 5), the majority of nodules (43.3%) were moderately hypoechoic. Isoechoic, hyperechoic and severely hypoechoic features had similar frequencies. A hypoechoic halo of the thyroid nodule was noted in 22 cases (7.3%).

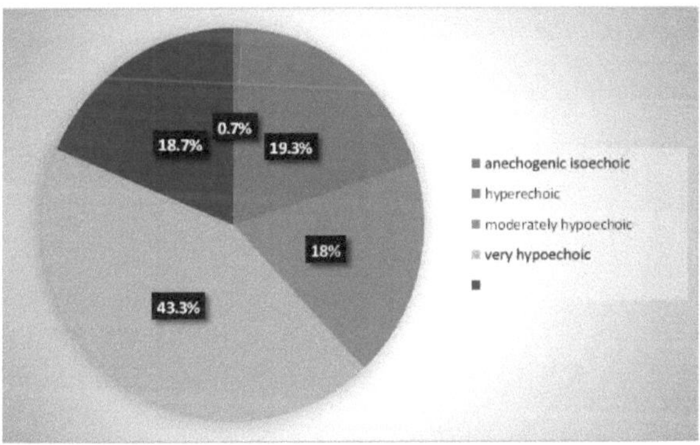

Figure 5: Echogenicity of thyroid nodules

Finally, according to the EU-TIRADS classification, the majority of nodules (39%) were considered EU-TIRADS 4 (Figure 6).

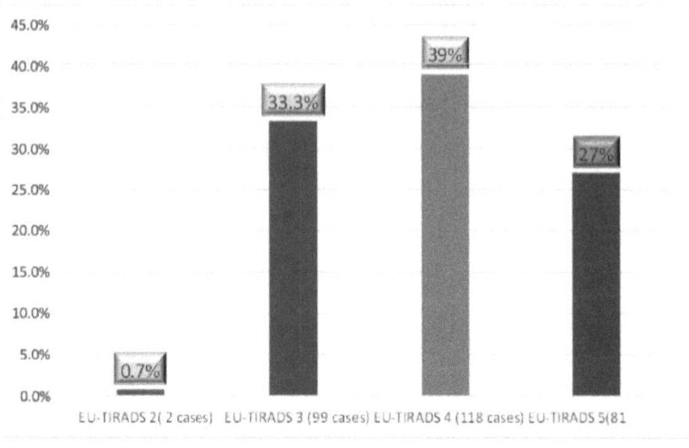

Figure 6: Distribution of patients according to EU-TIRADS classification

On clinical examination, seven patients (2.3%) had adenomegaly (Figure 7). The lymph node areas affected were II in 3 cases, III in 4 cases, IV in 2 cases and chain V in 2 cases.

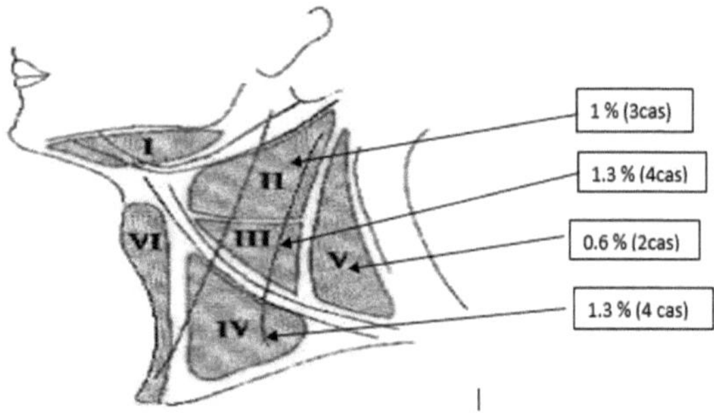

Figure 7: Ultrasound lymph node groups in adenomegaly

Table II: Ultrasound findings in thyroid nodules

		N	%
Nodules			
Nombre	Unique	129	43
	Multiple	171	57
Siège	Lobe droit	162	54
	Lobe gauche	137	45,7
	Isthme	1	0,3
Forme	Plus large que haut	269	89,6
	Plus haut que large	31	10,3
Échogénicité	Anéchogène	2	0.7
	Isoéchogène	58	19.3
	Hyperéchogène	54	18
	Modérément Hypoéchogène	130	43.3
	Fortement hypoéchogène	56	18.7
Limite inférieure	Plongeant	10	3,3
	Non plongeant	290	96,7
Vascularisation	Centrale	64	21,3
	Périphérique	140	46,7
	Mixte	96	32
Contours	Réguliers	242	80,6
	Irréguliers	58	19,3
Calcifications		136	45,33
Nature	Micro	58	19,3
	Macro	78	26

Nodules classified as EUTIRADS 3, i.e. isoechoic, were found in 33.3% of cases (Figure 8).

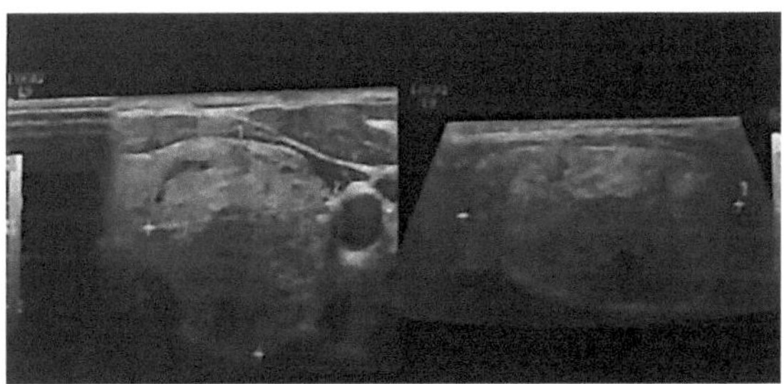

Figure 8: Isoechogenic heterogeneous oval-shaped left lobar nodule measuring 47*23*20 mm classified EUTIRADS 3.

Nodules classified as EUTIRADS 4, i.e. moderately hypoechoic, were in the majority in our study, being found in 39% of cases (Figure 9).

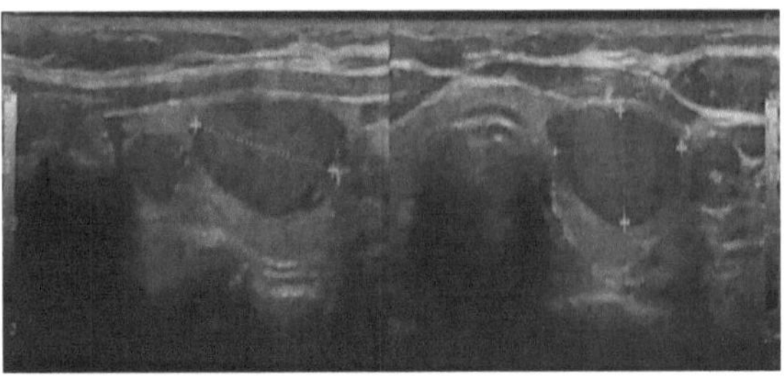

Figure 9: Moderately hypoechoic oval-shaped right lobar nodule classified as EUTIRADS 4

EUTIRADS 5 nodules were found in 27% of cases (Figure 10).

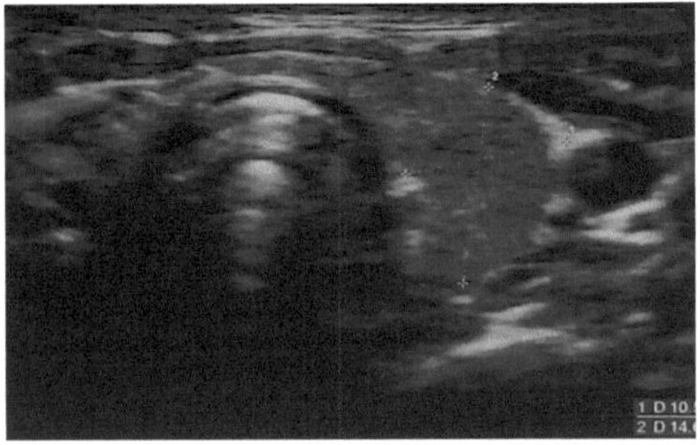

Figure 10: Heterogeneous isoechoic left lobar nodule of non-oval shape (taller than wide) containing microcalcifications classified as EUTIRADS 5.

1.3. Biological data

The thyroid work-up showed a:

- euthyroidism in 294 cases (98%);

- hypothyroidism in 3 cases (1%)

- hyperthyroidism in 3 cases (1%).

As for tumour markers, a thyrocalcitonin test was carried out in only one patient in our study, showing a high level of calcitonin.

Calcaemia was carried out in all cases and was normal.

1.4. Data from the cervico- thoracic CT scan

Cervico-thoracic CT scans were performed in 13 patients (4.3%) (when there was a doubt that 12 patients had a plunging tumour and 1 patient had a precessive adenopathy).

She revealed:

- A plunging character in 11 cases (84.6%) (extension into the anterior superior mediastinum in 9 cases and into the posterior superior mediastinum in 2 cases)
- Tracheal compression and deviation in 6 cases (46% of cases)
- Direct contact with vascular structures in 5 cases (38% of cases); direct contact with the aortic arch in 1 case, 2 cases of direct contact with the brachiocephalic arterial trunk and 3 with the brachiocephalic venous trunk.
- Oesophageal compression in 3 cases (23.07%)
- For the precessive adenopathy, the CT scan showed a jugulocarotid lymph node run with the presence of an adenopathy that comes into contact with the primary carotid artery while preserving the fatty border with infiltration of the pre-nodal fat associated with sub-centimetre spinal adenopathies.

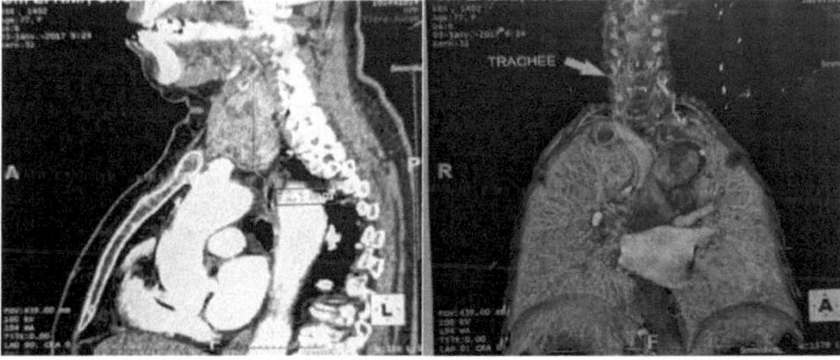

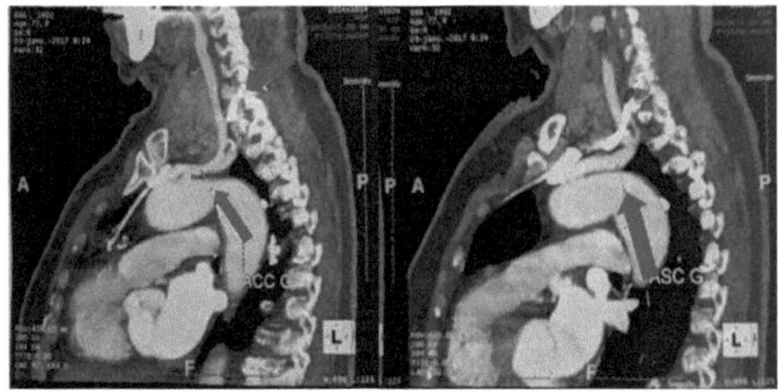

Figure 11: Cervico-thoracic CT scan in sagittal (a,c,d) and coronal (b) sections showing a goitre plunging at the expense of the left lobe of the thyroid gland (a) extending 2 cm beyond the upper edge of the sternum causing a lateral deviation to the right of the trachea (b) and the oesophagus resting inferiorly on the origin of the supra-aortic arterial trunks (d) and pushing the left common carotid artery to the left (c).

1.5. Data from thyroid scintigraphy

Only three patients had undergone thyroid scintigraphy (as part of a thyroid scan).the exploration of hyperthyroidism). It showed a hyperfixating goitre in 2 patients and a cold nodule in the remaining case.

1.6. Data from needle biopsy fine

Thyroid cytopunction was performed in 71 patients (23.67%) with a mean size of 22.16 mm (with extremes of 10 and 45 mm). We adopted the cytopunction recommendations published in the algorithm of the latest EUTIRADS 2017 classification (appendix 2). For the different punctured nodules in our study, the results met the Bethesda 2017 classification (appendix3) and were as follows (table III):

Table III: Breakdown of patients by cytopsy result

	Nombre des patients	Pourcentage
I-Non diagnostiqué	1	1,41
II-Bénin	8	11,27
III-atypies de signification indéterminée ou lésion folliculaire de signification indéterminée	21	29,58
IV-néoplasme folliculaire ou néoplasme folliculaire à cellules oncocytaires	16	22,54
V-lésions suspectes de malignité	15	21,16
VI-malin	10	14,08

The Bethesda classification data according to the EUTIRADS classification are detailed in Table IV :

EUTIRADS	Bethesda (annexe 3)	I	II	III	IV	V	VI	Non faite	Total
2	Effectif	0	0	0	0	0	0	2	2
	% par rapport aux cytoponctions faites	0	0	0	0	0	0		
3	Effectif	0	3	8	3	1	0	84	99
	% par rapport aux cytoponctions faites (n=15)	0	20	53,3	20	6,6	0		
4	Effectif	0	4	8	6	10	0	90	118
	% par rapport aux cytoponctions faites (n=28)	0	14,3	28,6	21,4	35,7	0		
5	Effectif	1	1	5	7	4	10	53	81
	% par rapport aux cytoponctions faites (n=28)	3,6	3,6	17,5	25	14,3	35,7		
Total		1	8	21	16	15	10	229	300

Table IV: Cytopsy results according to EUTIRADS classification

In addition, two patients underwent lymph node cytopuncture with thyroglobulin measurement in the cytopuncture fluid, and an elevated level was found in a single patient who was found to have lymph node metastasis from papillary thyroid carcinoma.

1.7. Surgical approach initial

We practised as an initial gesture:

- loboisthmectomy in 191 cases (63.7%);

- total thyroidectomy in 109 cases (36.3%);

- recurrent lymph node dissection in 115 cases (38.3%), uni and bilaterally in 53 (17.7%) and 62 (20.7%) cases respectively

- lateral lymph node dissection (groups II III IV) was performed in

7 cases (2.3%) due to the presence of adenomegaly associated with malignant nodules confirmed on extemporaneous examination, of which only one case was bilateral due to the presence of adenomegaly greater than 3 cm.

Extemporaneous examination showed the following results:

- Benin: 118 cases (39.3%)

- Waiting for definitive anatomopathological results (PFRA): 125 cases (41.7%)

- Malignant: 57 cases, i.e. 19% of cases.

1.8. Anatomopathological examination definitive

Anatomopathological examination revealed :

-Malignant lesions in 140 cases (46.7%), broken down as follows:

- papillary carcinoma in 130 cases (92.8%)

- vesicular carcinoma in 8 cases (5.7%)

- anaplastic carcinoma in 1 case (0.7%)

- medullary carcinoma in 1 case (0.7%)

-a benign lesion in 152 cases (50.7%) and

A non-invasive follicular thyroid neoplasm with nuclear characteristics of papillary carcinoma (NIFTP) in 8 cases (2.7%). The characteristics of malignant lesions are shown in Table V, including variants of papillary carcinoma.

Table V: Anatomopathological characteristics of malignant lesions

Number of Percentage

	patients	%
Capsular rupture	12	8,6
Vascular emboli	19	13,6
Recurrent lymph node metastasis	15	10,7
Lateral lymph node metastasis	2	1,42
Type		
Papillary carcinoma * Variants :	130	92,8
Papillary microcarcinoma	48	36,9
Vesicular	61	46,9
Oncocytic	11	8,5
Warthin-like	4	3,1
Cylindrical cell	2	1,5
Solid	2	1,5
High cell	2	1,5
Vesicular carcinoma	8	5,7
Anaplastic carcinoma	1	0,7
Medullary carcinoma	1	0.7

1.9.Surgical approach complementary

It was necessary to perform an additional procedure such as :

- total thyroidectomy in 73 patients (24.3%), 18 of whom had papillary microcarcinoma (multifocality in 12 patients, capsular rupture in 3 patients, tumour emboli in 3 patients);

- Totalization was accompanied by contralateral recurrential resection in all 73 patients.

1.10. Post- operative complications

The post-operative course was marked by the appearance of a thyroid compartment haematoma and wall suppuration in 1 (0.3%) and 2 (0.6%) cases respectively. Recurrent paralysis was noted in 20 patients, transient in 16 cases (5.3%) and permanent in 4 cases (0.13%). In addition, only one patient who had a lateral cut had a painful shoulder syndrome.

1.11. IRAtherapy and opotherapy substitutive

One hundred and twenty-five patients (41.7%) were treated with radio-active iodine during withdrawal. The average number of courses and iodine doses were 1.25±0.5 (1-4 courses) and ranged from 30 to 400 mCi (cumulative doses), respectively. The doses were delivered (table VI) according to the classification of the risk of relapse (low, medium and high risk) (appendix 4). Thirteen patients did not receive ARF therapy for papillary microcarcinoma unifocal with no lymph node metastases or distant metastases, pT1aN0M0. Treatment with L_thyroxine for frentive purposes was necessary in 140 patients (46.6%) and for replacement purposes in 41 cases (13.6%).

Table VI: Distribution of patients and doses of ARF therapy according to risk of relapse

	Nombre	Dose d'Irathérapie
Faible risque	40	Dose cumulée : 30-100 mci (30 mci/séance)
Risque Moyen	49	Dose cumulée : 100-200 mci (100mci/séance)
Haut risque	36	Dose cumulée : 100-400mci (100 mci /séance)

1.12. Post-operative chemotherapy / radiotherapy :

The patient, who had anaplastic carcinoma, was proposed for postoperative chemotherapy, but was subsequently lost to follow-up. The patient with a medullary carcinoma underwent postoperative radiotherapy following a lymph node recurrence that had been surgically resected.

1.13. Surveillance :

Our patients were monitored mainly clinically and biologically, with a A consultation every 3 months for the first year, then every 6 months. Sixty-eight patients were lost to follow-up, 12 of whom had been treated for thyroid cancer (including the patient with anaplastic cancer). TSH levels were checked in all our patients postoperatively and the dose of L_thyroxine was adjusted according to the target (frentive or substitutive dose).Thyroglobulin and anti-thyroglobulin antibodies were measured in patients treated for differentiated carcinoma: we had elevated thyroglobulin and anti-thyroglobulin antibody levels post irradiation in 20 patients, 6 of whom underwent repeat surgery for lymph node recurrence (papillary carcinoma initially classified as high risk) and 14 of whom underwent additional sessions of irradiation with subsequent normalisation of thyroglobulin and anti-thyroglobulin antibody values. Annual ultrasound monitoring was carried out systematically. for patients with carcinoma (n=140) and NIFTP (n=8). A follow-up ultrasound was performed despite a benign histology for patients who had undergone loboisthmectomy and in whom we suspected a nodule on the clinically remaining lobe (n=35). Calcitonin was measured postoperatively in a patient with medullary carcinoma. The level was elevated to 1200 ng/l in relation to a lateral lymph node recurrence, for which the patient underwent contralateral functional curage followed by postoperative radiotherapy.

2. Study analytical

2.1. Population: "Benin" and "Malin"

Initially we did not include in this study cases of anatomopathological lesion type NIFTP (N=8) A study association between the classification EU-TIRADS classification performed after cervical ultrasound and the anatomopathological results was carried out. The results were as follows (Table VII):

Table VII: Association between the EU-TIRADS classification and the study anatomopathological

Classification Pathological findings

	EU-TIRADS	Malin	Benin
2		0 (0%)	2 (1,3%)
3		31 (22,1%)	66 (43,4%)
4		58 (41,4%)	54 (35,5%)
5		51 (36,4%)	30 (19,7%)

2.1.1. Correlation between EU-TIRADS 3 score and pathological study

Ninety-seven patients (32.3% of the total population) had nodules classified as EU-TIRADS 3. They were confirmed as benign by pathological examination in the majority of cases (66/97 or 68%). This result was statistically significant (**$p<0.05$**) (Figure 12).

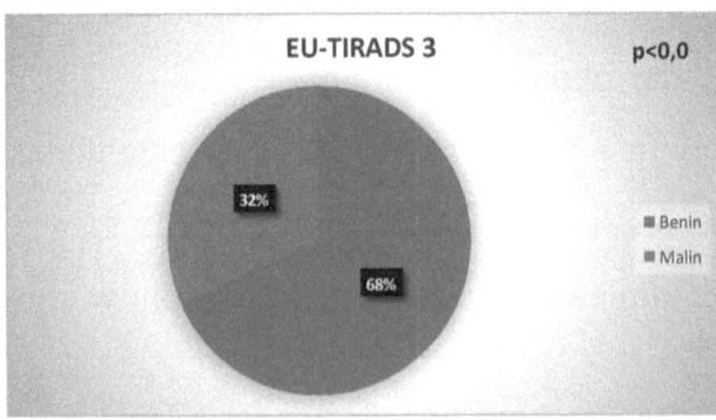

Figure 12: Distribution of EU-TIRADS 3 nodules according to anatomopathological result

The sensitivity and specificity of the EU-TIRADS 3 score were 22.1% and 55.9% with a PPV and NPV of 31.6% and 43.8%, respectively.

2.1.2. Relationship between the score EU-TIRADS SCORE 4 and anatomopathological study

In our population, 112 (37.33%) patients had nodules classified as EU- TIRADS 4.The number of benign and malignant lesions found on pathological examination was comparable, with 54 (48.2%) and 58 (51.7%) cases, respectively (p=0.249). The sensitivity and specificity of the EU-TIRADS 4 score were 41.4% and 65.1% with a PPV and NPV of 52.3% and 54.7%, respectively.

2.1.3. EU-TIRADS 5 score and anatomopathological study

Eighty-one (27.7%) patients had nodules classified as EU-TIRADS 5. A On anatomopathological study, 30 (37%) nodules were benign and 51 (63%) malignant.The sensitivity and specificity of the EU-TIRADS 5 score were 36.4% and 80.3% with a PPV and NPV of 63% and 57.8%, respectively. A statistical association in favour of malignancy was determined between the EU-TIRADS 5 score and the pathological study, with a significant difference **(p=0.001)**.

We also studied the association between the pathological findings and the various ultrasound criteria defining the EU-TIRADS 5 class (table VIII). Only irregular contours and high hypoechogenicity were significantly more common in malignant lesions, with sensitivity and specificity of 62% and 85.2% for irregular contours, respectively, and 76.5% and 43.3% for high hypoechogenicity, respectively. The two remaining ultrasound features, microcalcifications and non-oval shape, had sensitivities and specificities of 78.4% and 40% and 35.4% and 62%, respectively (Table IX).

Table VIII: Association between EU-TIRADS 5 ultrasound signs and anatomopathological study

Signes échographiques	Résultats anatomopathologiques		P
	Malin	Bénin	
Contours irréguliers	31 (60,8%)	4 (13,33%)	<0,01
Nodule fortement hypoéchogène	39 (76,5%)	17 (56,7%)	0,049
microcalcifications	40 (78,4%)	18 (60%)	0,076
Forme non ovale	17 (33,3%)	11 (36,7%)	0,824

Table IX: Sensitivity and specificity of EU-TIRADS 5 ultrasound signs

Signes échographiques	Sensibilité	spécificité
Contours irréguliers	85,2 %	43.3 %
Nodule fortement hypoéchogène	62 %	76.5 %
microcalcifications	87,4 %	40 %
Forme non ovale	35,4 %	62 %

We then studied the impact of the association of ultrasound criteria on the risk of malignancy, and found that the association of more than two criteria was associated with the highest percentage of malignancy, which was 86.7% (table X),As for the different types of association of the ultrasound criteria, in our study, the different combinations of criteria were characterised by a high percentage of malignancy with a rate that varied between 81 and 96%. The association of hypoechogenicity and microcalcifications represented the association most statistically related to malignancy (Table X).

Table X: Impact of the combination of EU-TIRADS 5 ultrasound criteria on the risk of malignancy

EUTIRADS 5 nodule	Number	Malignant anatomopathological examination
A single criterion	20 (24,7%)	6(30%)
Two criteria	31(38.3%)	19(61,3%)
>two criteria	30(37%)	26(86,7%)

Table XI: Relationship between malignancy and different combinations of criteria of EUTIRADS 5

Nodule EUTIRADS 5	Nombre	Examen anatomopathologique malin
Hypoéchogénicité +contours irréguliers	26 (32,1%)	24(92,3%)
Hypoéchogénicité +microcalcifications	37(45,7%)	30(81,1%)
Contours irréguliers +microcalcifications	25(30,9%)	24(96%)

We found that the percentage prediction of malignancy decreased with increasing nodule size. For nodules larger than 30 mm, the percentage was only 30% compared with 100% for nodules smaller than 10 mm (table XII).

Table XII: EU-TIRADS 5 score prediction of malignancy according to nodular size (threshold 30mm)

Nodule size	Number	Malignant anatomopathological examination
< 10 mm	7 (8,6%)	7(100%)
10 - 30 mm	54(66,7%)	38(70,4%)
>30 mm	20(24,7%)	6(30%)

2.2. Population: Benin, Malin and NIFTP

In our total population, eight cases of NIFTP-type lesions were identified. In a second phase, we carried out the same analytical study as for the 2.1.on the one hand on the population: "Benin+NIFTP" versus "Malin", on the other hand on the population: "Malin+NIFTP" versus "Benin" and we have drawn the same conclusions.This anatomopathological entity "NIFTP", whether added to the "Benin" or "Malin" groups, had not changed the results compared with analysis that did not include NIFTP ($p = 0.723$), tables XIII and XIV. Six of the 8 cases were classified as EU-TIRADS 4, while the remaining 2 were EU-TIRADS 3.

Table XIII: Association between EUTIRADS 2017 classification and the study anatomopathology, including NIFTP in malignancy

Classification EUTIRADS	Résultats histologiques		Total
	Malin (+NIFTP)	Bénin	
2	0	2 (1,31%)	
3	33 (22,3 %)	66 (43,4%)	
4	64 (43,2 %)	54 (35,5%)	
5	51 (34,45 %)	30 (19,7%)	
Total	148	152	300

Table XIV: Association between EUTIRADS 2017 classification and the study anatomopathology including NIFTP in benignity

Classification EUTIRADS	Résultats histologiques		Total
	Malin	Bénin (+NIFTP)	
2	0	2 (1,35%)	
3	31 (22,1 %)	68 (42,5%)	
4	58 (41,4 %)	60 (37,5%)	
5	51 (36,4 %)	30 (18,75%)	
Total	140	160	300

DISCUSSION

1. Main results :

We conducted a monocentric retrospective study in the ENT and CCF department of the Mohamed Taher Maâmouri Nabeul hospital that included 300 patients with thyroid nodular pathology operated on in our department during a 3-year period from July 2017 to July 2020. The mean age of the patients was 47.04 years [extremes 10 years and 78 years]. A clear female predominance was noted with a sex ratio of 0.1. The average consultation time was 10 months. Anterior basicervical swelling was the most frequent reason for consultation, associated with dysphagia in 8% of cases, dyspnoea in 2.7% and dysphonia in 0.7%. The anterior basicervical swelling was firm and mobile on swallowing in 94 of cases, associated with homolateral adenomegaly in 2.3% of cases, only one patient presented with immobility of the vocal cord homolateral to the nodule. On cervical ultrasound, the mean size of the nodules was 28.83 mm with extremes ranging from 0.5 to 67 mm, 57% of our patients had a multinodular goitre, plunging in 3.3% of cases, the most frequent location was mediolobar followed by the upper pole. The majority of nodules were moderately hypoechoic (43.3%), with similar frequencies of isoechoic, hyperechoic and severely hypoechoic features. Nodules were classified as EUTIRADS 2, 3, 4 and 5 in 0.7%, 33.3%, 39% and 27% of cases respectively. According to the clinical examination, seven patients (2.3%) had adenopathy. The lymph node areas involved were III+IV in 2 cases and II+III, II+V, III, IV and II+IV+V in 1 case each. Cervicothoracic CT scans were performed in 13 patients, and were pathological in 11. Fine needle cytopuncture was performed in 71 patients (23.6%), according to the 2017 Bethesda classification, the punctured nodules were classified as Bethesda I,II,III,IV,V and VI in 1.41%, 11.27% ,29.58%, 22.54%,21.1%+ and 14.08% respectively. As first-line surgery, our patients underwent loboisthmectomy in 191 (63.7%) cases, total thyroidectomy in 108 cases (36%), recurrent lymph node dissection in 115 cases (38.3%), and lateral lymph node dissection in 7 cases (2.3%), only one of which was bilateral. Extemporaneous examination showed benign tumours in 118 cases (39.3%), awaiting definitive anatomopathological result (PFAR) in 125 cases (41.7%) and malignancy in 57 cases (19%). The definitive anatomopathological examination revealed malignant lesions in 140 cases (46.7%), of which papillary carcinoma accounted for 91.4% of cases, followed by vesicular carcinoma in 5.7% of cases, with one case of medullary carcinoma and one case of anaplastic carcinoma. One hundred and fifty-two patients had benign lesions (50.7 %) and only 8 cases of NIFTP-type lesions (2.7%). In 73 patients (24.3% of cases) it was necessary to perform an additional procedure such as total thyroidectomy combined with contralateral recurrential curage. The post-operative course was marked by the appearance of a haematoma of the thyroid compartment and suppuration of the wall in 1 (0.3%) and 2 (0.6%) cases respectively. Recurential paralysis was noted in 20 patients, transient in 16 (5.3%) and permanent in 4 (0.13%). In addition, only one patient who had a lateral cut had a painful shoulder syndrome. Complementary treatment with ARF therapy was necessary in 125 patients (41.7%). Substitutive opotherapy was indicated in 41 patients and was effective in 140 cases (53%).A statistical study was carried out to compare the ultrasound data (EUTIRADS 2017 classification) with the definitive histological results. At the end of the analytical study, we found malignancy prediction percentages of 0%, 22.1%, 41.4% and 36.4% for nodules classified as EUTIRADS 2, 3, 4 and 5 respectively. Nodules classified as EUTIRADS 3 had a sensitivity, specificity PPV and NPV of 22.1%, 55.9%, 31.6% and 43.8% respectively, with a significant p-value ($p<0.01$). Nodules classified as EUTIRADS 4 had a sensitivity and specificity of 41.4% and 65.1% with a PPV and NPV of 52.3% and 54.7%, respectively, and a non-significant p-value (0.249). Nodules classified as EUTIRADS 5 had a sensitivity and specificity of 36.4% and 80.3% with a PPV and NPV of 63% and 57.8%, respectively. A statistical association in favour of malignancy was determined between the EU-

TIRADS 5 score and the pathological study, with a significant difference **(p=0.001)**. We also studied the association between the pathological findings and the various ultrasound criteria defining the EU-TIRADS 5 class. Only irregular contours and high hypoechogenicity were significantly more common in malignant lesions, with sensitivity and specificity of 62% and 85.2% and 76.5% and 43.3%, respectively. In addition, we found that the association of more than two criteria had a percentage of malignancy than in the case of the presence of a single criterion, which was 86.7%. The association of hypoechogenicity and microcalcifications was more significantly related to malignancy. We carried out the same analytical study on the "Benign+NIFTP" versus "Malignant" population and the : "Malin+NIFTP" versus "Benin" and this entity did not change the results.

2. Strengths and weaknesses of the study :

2.1. Limitations of our study :

2.1.1. Retrospective nature of the study

Our work was a retrospective study, spread over 3 years. The retrospective nature of the study means that there may be a lack of data in the files. Nevertheless, the missing data were deemed to have a minor impact on the results.

2.1.2. Selection bias :

Only operated nodules were included and the ultrasound risk of malignancy is relatively higher compared with a sample including all nodules.Our population was essentially from the North-East region and was therefore not representative of all the regions of Tunisia. This is explained by the sectorisation of healthcare use by region.On the other hand, the ultrasound scans were not performed by the same radiologist, with a risk of inter-observer variability in the assessment of thyroid nodules.

2.2. The strengths of our study :

2.2.1. Sample size :

Our study included 300 patients over a period of 3 years. It is therefore one of the largest series in our country over this short period.

2.2.2. Accuracy of valuation :

We compared the various EUTIRADS ultrasound classes with the results of the definitive histological examination, as well as the various EUTIRADS 5 criteria and their associations, enabling a precise assessment of the diagnostic performance of ultrasound.

3. EUTIRADS 2017 classification and prediction of malignancy :

3.1. EUTIRADS 2017 classification reminder :

In 2017, the European Association of Endocrinology (ETA) proposed to create new guidelines and published a new simplified TIRADS, which is called EUTIRADS for 'European - Thyroid Imaging and Reporting Data System' with the same aim of improving interobserver reproducibility and simplifying the communication of results.

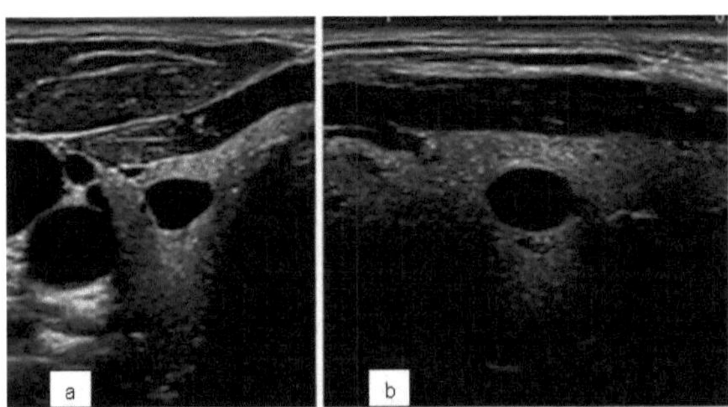

EUTIRADS 2 :a/ Transverse section and b/ Longitudinal section [9] Pure anechogenic cyst

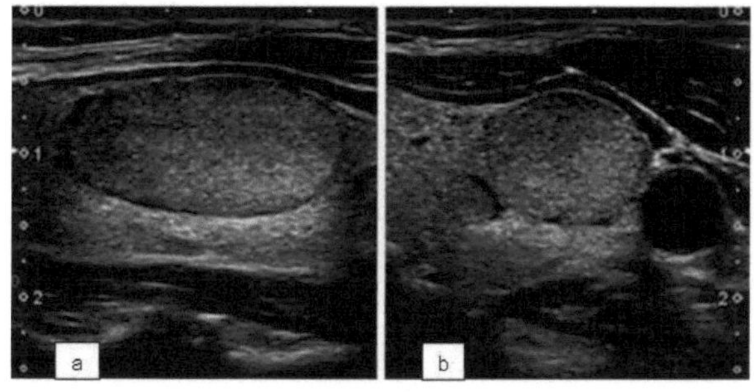

EUTIRADS 3 :a/ Longitudinal section. b/ Cross-section [9].

Low-risk isoechoic nodule with oval shape and smooth margins without high-risk features

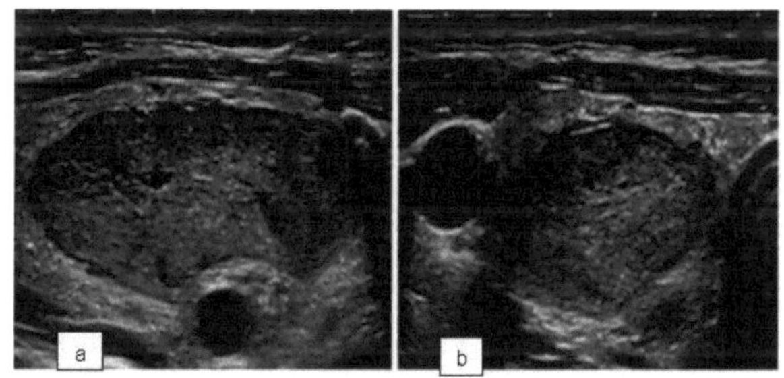

EUTIRADS 4 : a/Longitudinal section. b/Cross-section [9].

Slightly hypoechoic nodule with an oval shape and regular borders, with no high-risk features.

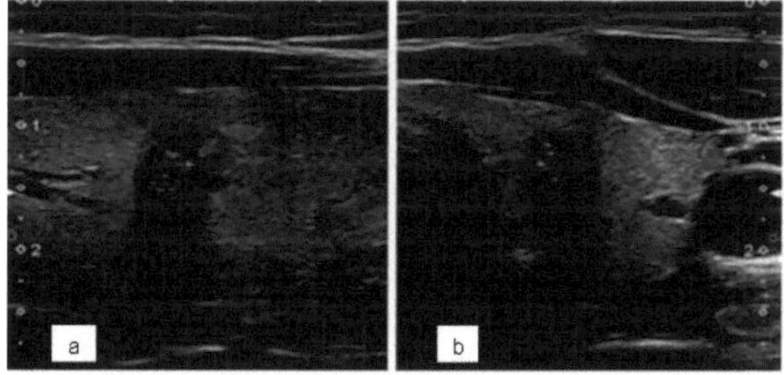

EUTIRADS 5 : a/ Longitudinal section. b/ Transverse section[9].

High-risk nodule with non-oval shape, speculated margins, microcalcifications and marked hypo-echogenicity *marked hypoechogenicity: darker than surrounding muscles; suspicious shape: not oval (taller than wide or round); irregular margins including microlobulated, spiculated and suggestive of extrathyroidal extension; microcalcifications: calcifications about 1 mm in size without posterior shadow located in the solid component of a nodule)[10].

3.2. Risk of malignancy and EUTIRADS classification :

In our series, benign nodules were observed in 152 patients and malignant nodules in 140 patients. Several series have examined the reliability of the EUTIRADS classification in predicting malignancy: A prospective study by Roussanka [11] investigating the performance of the EUTIRADS classification in predicting malignancy in 783 thyroid nodules showed a malignancy rate of 0% in category 2, 0% in category 3, 3.8% in category 4 and 30.6% in category 5. [11] In our study the risk of malignancy for each category was 0%. 22%, 41% and 36% for scores 2, 3, 4 and 5 respectively. Our results are consistent with those found in other series [12] [13]. [14] and [15], regarding the higher-than-recommended malignancy rate in EUTIRADS 3 (> 3%) and EUTIRADS 4 (> 17 %). As for the EUTIRADS 5 category, our results are consistent with those of Hasnaoui [15], Roussanka [11] and Dobruch-sobrzack [16] with a rate close to the lower limit of the European Thyroid Association guidelines (26%) [9]. However, among these different studies, we found those which reported a malignancy rate for category 5 close to the upper limit of the guidelines, some exceeding this limit (86%) [12-14] (The results of the different series are summarised in Table XV).

Table XV: Risk of malignancy according to the EUTIRADS classification

Score EUTIRADS	Risque de malignité %							
	Filali et al [12]	Hasnaoui et al [15]	Castellana et al [14]	Roussanka et al[11]	Chatti et al [13]	Dobruch-Sobczak et al [16]	Myzia et al[17]	Notre série
EUTIRADS 2	0 %	2.27 %	0.5 %	0 %	0 %	0 %	0 %	0 %
EUTIRADS 3	20 %	7.18 %	5.9 %	0%	15.6 %	3 %	12 %	22,1%
EUTIRADS 4	31.25 %	7.4 %	21.4 %	3.8 %	69 %	19 %	35 %	41%
EUTIRADS 5	100 %	30.4 %	76.1 %	30.6 %	76.9 %	43 %	53 %	35 %

In our study, the sensitivity, specificity, PPV and NPV were 77%, 69%, 56% and 69% respectively. These results show a lower sensitivity than in the literature, which means that there is a higher percentage of false negatives. These data may be explained by the fact that thyroid ultrasound in our study was performed by different radiologists with different experience some of whom were new to the EUTIRADS 2017 score and therefore increased inter-observer variability. Our results are similar to those found by Hasnaoui and chatti [13,15] (table XVI).

Table XVI: Comparison between the results of our series and those of the literature regarding the diagnostic performance of the EUTIRADS system

Série / Score EUTIRADS	Roussanka et al [11]	Filali et al [12]	Hasnaoui et al[15]	Castellana et al [14]	Chatti et al [13]	Notre série
Sensibilité	91.3 %	87%	76 %	83.5 %	60 %	77 %
Spécificité	74.6 %	83%	62 %	84.3 %	82 %	69 %
VPP	30.6 %	73 %	26 %	76.1 %	77 %	56%
VPN	98.6 %	92 %	93 %	85.4 %	67 %	69%

Sillery et al and kovatcheva et al have shown in their studies of the sonographic aspects of thyroid carcinoma that the suspicious sonographic features assessed in EU-TIRADS are highly specific for papillary thyroid carcinoma, but are not validated for follicular thyroid cancer, which often has a low-risk sonographic appearance[11,18]. There are differing views regarding the ability of TIRADS to recognise follicular carcinomas. The American Thyroid Association (ATA) considers that follicular carcinomas less than 20 mm in greatest diameter may not be recognised because distant metastases rarely occur in such lesions[19].

Solimosy et al found no significant difference between papillary thyroid carcinoma (PTC) and medullary thyroid carcinoma (MTC) in the presence of suspicious ultrasound features and verified that the performance of EU-TIRADS in the diagnosis of MTC is as good as in PTC[20,21] . Yan Shen et al demonstrated that EUTIRADS has the best diagnostic efficiency, with the highest sensitivity, PPV and accuracy for the identification of medullary carcinoma (61.8%, 75.0% and 79.2%, respectively)[22] .

Several authors have compared the different TIRADS systems, and T.XU et al [23] have shown that EU-TIRADS has a higher reproducibility than ACR-TIRADS and KSThR-TIRADS, probably due to a higher number of TIRADS tests. lower level of highly suspicious features and a more progressive score [23]. Koc et al showed that EUTIRADS had a better sensitivity (86.7%) than the other scores (ACR, KSTHR), especially for nodules smaller than 10 mm [24]. However, Zhe Jin et al [25] demonstrated that EUTIRADS had a lower sensitivity and discrimination percentage than C-TIRADs and ACR- TIRADS and a specificity similar to C TIRADs [25].

Nodule size has been shown to have an impact on the performance of EU-TIRADS in predicting malignancy[26-28]. Specificity, PPV and accuracy were significantly better for nodules ≥ 10 mm [11,28,29]. Myzia et al showed that the diagnostic performance of the EUTIRADS score and the Bethesda classification regressed for nodules larger than 3 cm [17]. In our study we found a better performance of the EUTIRADS score for lesions smaller than 3 cm with a malignancy rate varying between 70 and 100%, and a decrease in performance for lesions larger than 3 cm as demonstrated by Myzia et al[18]. It has also been shown that the best predictor of the risk of malignancy is nodule elasticity, so the lack of inclusion of elasticity in the EU-TIRADS score could be considered one of the limitations of this classification[16].

Gerdi_ Tuli et al studied the performance of the EUTIRADS system on thyroid nodules in the paediatric population and found that the diagnosis of cancer was missed in 26.9% of cases[30]. Furthermore, Sema Hepsen et al [31] demonstrated that the association of subacute thyroiditis could erroneously affect the EUTIRADS score due to the inhomogeneous and ill-defined hypoechoic areas caused by thyroiditis. It has been recommended that repeat ultrasonography should be performed after an episode of subacute thyroiditis to improve the performance of the EUTIRADS score[31].

Szczepanek-Parulska et al [32] published a recent experimental prospective study on 133 thyroid nodules in which they studied the performance of Computer Aided Diagnosis (S-Detect) in detecting malignancy and compared its results with those of EUTIRADS. The aim of this new complementary examination is to reduce or even eliminate inter-observer variability in order to increase diagnostic accuracy, particularly when the examination is carried out by radiologists outside reference centres for the diagnosis of thyroid cancer. This study demonstrated a high sensitivity of S-Detect (89.4%), comparable to the assessment made by experienced sonographers using the EU-TIRADS scale (90.9), the specificity of S-Detect (80.6%) was also fairly high and better than that of experienced sonographers (61.2%)[32]. They also studied the combination of S-Detect with EUTIRADS and concluded that the combined model taking into account both S-Detect and EU-TIRADS assessment is better than either approach alone[32].

3.3. Correlation between different EUTIRADS 2017 scores and pathological findings :

3.3.1. Correlation between EUTIRADS II and pathological examination :

Due to insufficient numbers (2 cases), we have not analysed this correlation.

in our study. In fact, half of the false negatives in the TIRADS classification are presented by predominantly cystic nodules (EUTIRADS2), which also represent 1-3% of thyroid carcinomas and in most cases are papillary carcinomas of classical variant with a strong cystic component. In these cases, the association of hypoechogenicity and/or microcalcifications should draw attention to a risk of malignancy. Cytopuncture, if performed, should involve the solid component to be more contributory[33].

3.3.2. Correlation between EUTIRADS III and pathological examination :

The risk of malignancy for nodules classified as EUTIRADS 3 varied between 3 and 4% in the guidelines[9]. In our study it represented 22%, our results are relatively higher than the theoretical values but are in line with the results of Shi et al [34] and Chatti et al [13], which can be explained in part by the sample, which only included patients who had undergone surgery. Dobruch-Sobczak K et al [16] demonstrated an inversely proportional relationship between lesion size and the risk of malignancy for EU-TIRADS 3 nodules [16].

Hyperechoic nodules are characterised by being rich in colloid and poor in cells. This reassuring feature is rarely malignant; the risk of malignancy varies from 1 to 5% [35,36]. One to three per cent of thyroid carcinomas are solid nodules Isoechogenic nodules (EUTIRADS3) are usually known to be at low risk of malignancy. This entity accounts for half of the TIRADS false negatives[33], and isoechoic nodules are associated with a variable risk of malignancy ranging from 12% to 26% [37]. Leenhardt has shown that this risk is reduced to 7% if the nodules are surrounded by a clear peripheral halo[35].

Follicular variant papillary carcinomas are the most affected by these false negatives, followed to a lesser extent by follicular carcinomas. [9,38] In fact, carcinomas are isoechoic in 15% of cases, but mostly associated with other signs of strong suspicion such as spiculated margins and non-oval shape. [39]

Compared with DTC, follicular carcinomas are more frequently iso or hypoechoic, non-calcified but round in shape with regular margins[37,40]. These characteristics distinguish them sonographically from follicular adenomas. This calls into question the fact that the distinction between follicular adenoma and follicular carcinoma is only histological[20].

3.3.3. Correlation between EUTIRADS IV and anatomopathological examination :

The risk of malignancy for nodules classified as EUTIRADS IV varies between 6 and 17% in the guidelines[9]. In our study, this risk was estimated at 41%, close to those found by FILALI et al (31%) and Myzia et al (35%). These higher figures can probably be explained by the fact that the sample included only patients who had undergone surgery. Maino et al[41] reported that EU-TIRADS 4 was unable to predict malignancy. On the other hand, Roussanka et al, Tugendsam et al and Ha et al [11,42,43] demonstrated in their studies that the prevalence of moderate hypoechogenicity was similar in benign and malignant lesions [11,42,43]. However, Kovatcheva et al[11] have shown that the diagnostic value of moderate hypoechogenicity, as a single EUTIRADS 4 marker of malignancy, is insufficient and considered that it should be supported by additional ultrasound features, such as vascularity or elasticity. Our study is in line with the results of the literature: we found no statistically significant relationship between the EUTIRADS 4 score and the anatomopathological result.

3.3.4. Correlation between EUTIRADS V and pathological examination :

The risk of malignancy for nodules classified as EUTIRADS V varies between 26 and 87% according to the guidelines [9]. We found an estimated rate of 35% in our series comparable to that found by Hasnaoui et al and Roussanka et al [11,15].

With regard to marked hypoechogenicity, the results in the literature vary between authors, especially concerning the sensitivity of this feature, with results ranging from 80 to 93.9% [16]. In our study, the sensitivity of marked hypoechogenicity was low (62%). In addition, most authors agree on a low specificity of 27% to 40%[16,44] and a low PPV of 24% for this feature[44], as some benign lesions may present as strongly hypoechoic nodules.Strong hypoechogenicity was noted in 76.5% of malignant nodules in our series compared with 56% of benign nodules, with a statistically significant difference ($p = 0.049$). Irregular margins have been identified by most authors as one of the most critical criteria for malignancy. It has been observed in 50 to 75% of cancers in the various studies (62% in our study, $p<0.01$) with a high specificity of >85% [45,46].

We found a specificity of 43.3% for this criterion, close to the result noted by Remonti et al = 50.5% [47], but the sensitivity of this characteristic was high in our study = 85.2%. Non-oval nodules have been associated with malignancy in 50-70% of cases [48,49] in the literature, compared with 33.3% in our study. This criterion has been considered particularly highly specific by some authors[16], compared with a moderate specificity of 62% in our study. Microcalcifications have been noted in more than 80% of cancers [50,51], a figure comparable to our series which found 78.4% microcalcifications in malignant nodules (but in our study the difference with benign nodules was not statistically significant), contrary to the authors [50,51]. Liénart et al [50] and Frates et al [52] have shown that the presence of microcalcifications increases the risk of malignancy by 2.5

As for the combination of EUTIRADS 5 ultrasound criteria, Peccin et al [44] showed that 80% of malignant cases had four or more positive features. The sensitivity and specificity of ultrasound diagnosis considering more than four features were 80% and 100% respectively, with a PPV of 100% and an NPV of 95.5% [44]. In our study, patients with more than two features had a higher percentage of malignancy (86.7%) compared to patients with only one feature (30%) with a sensitivity of 96%. Remonti et al [47] found that the specificity of microcalcifications, irregular margins, non oval shape and marked hypoechogenicity to distinguish benign from malignant nodules was 39.5%, 50.5, 96.6 and 62.3%, respectively. However, the reported sensitivity of the aforementioned criteria in the same study was 87.8, 83.1, 26.7 and 62.7%, respectively.[47]

In our study, irregular contours and high hypoechogenicity were significantly more common in malignant lesions. For irregular contours, the sensitivity and specificity were 82% and 43.3% respectively. For severe hypoechogenicity, sensitivity and specificity were 62% and 76.5% respectively. For microcalcifications, sensitivity was 87.4% and specificity 40%. For the non-oval form, sensitivity and specificity were 35.4% and 62% respectively. We also found that the association of irregular contours with microcalcifications and the association of irregular contours with hypoechogenicity were the most predictive of malignancy with percentages of 92.3% and 96% respectively.

Table XVII: Diagnostic performance of the various EUTIRADS criteria V

Critère	Remonti et al [47] Sensibilité Spécificité		Roussanka et al [11] Sensibilité Spécificité		Notre série Sensibilité Spécificité	
Forte Hypoéchogénicité	62.7 %	62.3 %	72 %	50 %	62 %	76.5%
Contours irréguliers	83.1 %	50.5%	64 %	48 %	85.2%	43.3%
Microcalcification	87.8 %	39.5 %	74 %	50 %	78.4%	40 %
Forme non ovale	26.7%	96.6 %	77 %	54 %	35.4%	62%

CONCLUSIONS

Issues :

Thyroid nodules are a frequent clinical and radiological entity, most of which are benign. However, advances in ultrasound have been associated with over-diagnosis of malignant nodules. Ultrasound and cytopuncture are the initial diagnostic pairing in the management of thyroid nodules. For this reason, several learned societies in endocrinology and radiology have established radiological scores based on the ultrasound criteria most likely to be malignant, in order to stratify the risk of malignancy of a thyroid nodule, have a standardised ultrasound lexicon and codify management. Among these ultrasound classifications, EU-TIRADS 2017 is the most recent and the one used in Tunisia. The aim of our study was to evaluate the diagnostic performance of the EUTIRADS 2017 classification by confirming it with the results of the definitive histology. To this end, we conducted a retrospective study in the Department of Otolaryngology and Head and Neck Surgery at the Mohamed Taher Maâmouri University Hospital in Nabeul on 300 patients who underwent thyroid surgery for nodular pathology and were managed in our department over a 3-year period from July 2017 to July 2020. Epidemiologically, the mean age of patients was 47.04 years [range 16-78 years]. There was a clear predominance of females, with a sex ratio of 0.1. The average consultation time was 10 months. Anterior basicervical swelling was the most frequent reason for consultation, associated with dysphagia in 8% of cases, dyspnoea in 2.7% and dysphonia in 0.7%. The anterior basicervical swelling was firm and mobile on swallowing in 90 of cases, associated with homolateral adenomegaly in 2.3% of cases, only one patient presented with immobility of the vocal cord homolateral to the nodule. On cervical ultrasound, the mean size of the nodules was 28.83 mm, and 57% of our patients had a multinodular goitre, which plunged in 3.3% of cases. The majority of nodules were moderately hypoechoic (43.3%), with similar frequencies of isoechoic, hyperechoic and severely hypoechoic features. Nodules were classified as EUTIRADS 2, 3, 4 and 5 in 0.7%, 33.3%, 39% and 27% of cases respectively. According to the clinical examination, seven patients (2.3%) had adenopathy. The lymph nodes affected were III+IV in 2 cases and II+III, II+V, III, IV and II+IV+V in 1 case each. Cervicothoracic CT scans were performed in 13 patients, and were pathological in 11 cases. Fine needle aspiration was performed in 71 patients (23.6%), according to the 2017 Bethesda classification, the nodules punctured were classified as Bethesda I,II,III,IV,V and VI in 1.41%, 11.27% ,29.58%, 22.54%,21,1+ and 14.08% respectively. As initial surgery, our patients underwent loboisthmectomy in 191 (63.7%) cases, total thyroidectomy in 108 cases (36%), recurrent lymph node dissection in 115 cases (38.3%), and lateral lymph node dissection in 7 cases (2.3%), only one of which was bilateral. The final anatomopathological examination revealed malignant lesions in 140 cases (46.7%), of which papillary carcinoma accounted for 91.4% of cases, followed by vesicular carcinoma in 5.7% of cases, with one case of medullary carcinoma and one case of anaplastic carcinoma. One hundred and fifty-two patients had a benign lesion (50.7%) and only 8 cases of NIFT lesion (2.7%). It was necessary to perform an additional procedure such as total thyroidectomy combined with recurrent curage in 73 patients (24.3% of cases). Complementary treatment with ARF therapy was required for 125 patients (41.7%). Substitutive opotherapy was indicated in 37 patients and was effective in 140 cases (53%).A statistical study was carried out to compare the ultrasound data (EUTIRADS 2017 classification) with the definitive histological results. At the end of the analytical study, we found a percentage prediction of malignancy of 0%, 22.1%, 41.4% and 36.4% for nodules classified as EUTIRADS 2, 3, 4 and 5 respectively. Nodules classified as EUTIRADS 3 had a se, sp, VPP and VPN of 22.1%, 55.9%, 31.6% and 43.8% respectively with a significant p-value ($p<0.01$). Nodules classified as EUTIRADS 4 had an se and sp of 41.4% and 65.1% with a PPV and NPV of 52.3% and 54.7%, respectively, and a non-significant p value (0.249). Nodules classified as EUTIRADS 5 had a sensitivity and specificity of 36.4% and 80.3% with a PPV and NPV of 63% and 57.8%, respectively. A statistical association in favour of malignancy was determined between the EU-TIRADS 5 score and the pathology study, with a significant difference (**p=0.001**). We then studied the association between the anatomical and pathological results. pathological lesions and the various ultrasound criteria defining the EU- TIRADS 5 class. Irregular contours and strong hypoechogenicity were significantly more noted in malignant lesions, with a sensitivity and specificity of 85.2% and 43.3% for irregular contours and a sensitivity and specificity of 62 and 76.5% for strong hypoechogenicity. In addition, the association of more than two criteria was found to have the highest percentage of malignancy at 86.7%. The association of hypoechogenicity and microcalcifications was characterised by the most significant P. We carried out the same analytical study on the "Benin+NIFTP" versus "Malignant" population and the "Malignant+NIFTP" versus "Benin" population and this entity did not change the results. In the light of our results and by analysing those of the literature, we conclude that the EUTIRADS 2017 classification is of considerable help in the detection of thyroid cancers, particularly via the criteria of the EUTIRADS V score, which have proved to be highly sensitive and/or specific.We consider that this classification remains valid and reliable with certain additions, namely the study of elasticity and vascularity for the EUTIRADS 4 score, and consideration of the number of malignancy criteria for the EUTIRADS 5 score. The reliability of this classification is improved by combining it with cytological studies. and above all molecular tests. In the coming years, we hope to optimise the prediction of thyroid malignancy using computer-assisted ultrasound diagnosis.

REFERENCES

1. Wémeau JL, Sadoul JL, D'herbomez M, Monpeyssen H, Tramalloni J, Leteurtre E, et al. Recommendations of the French Society of Endocrinology for the management of thyroid nodules. Presse Med. Sept 2011;40(9):793-826.

2. Shayganfar A, Hashemi P, Esfahani MM, Ghanei AM, Moghadam NA, Ebrahimian

S. Prediction of thyroid nodule malignancy using thyroid imaging reporting and data system (TIRADS) and nodule size. Clin Imaging. 2020 Apr;60(2):222-7.

3. Horvath E, Silva CF, Majlis S, Rodriguez I, Skoknic V, Castro A, et al. Prospective validation of the ultrasound based TIRADS (thyroid imaging reporting and data system) classification: results in surgically resected thyroid nodules. Eur Radiol. 2017 Jun;27(6):2619-28.

4. Smith Bindman R, Lebda P, Feldstein VA, Sellami D, Goldstein RB, Brasic N, et al. Risk of thyroid cancer based on thyroid ultrasound imaging characteristics: results of a population-based study. JAMA Intern Med. 2013 Oct;173(19):1788- 96.

5. Durante C, Costante G, Lucisano G, Bruno R, Meringolo D, Paciaroni A, et al. The natural history of benign thyroid nodules. J Am Med Assoc. 2015 Mar;313(9):926-35.

6. Patel N, Stechman MJ. Management of the thyroid nodule. Surgery. 2020 Nov;38(12):786-93.

7. Haute Autorité de Santé. Investigation of thyroid pathologies in adults: relevance and quality criteria for ultrasound, relevance of ultrasound-guided cytopuncture [Online]. Sept 2021 [Accessed 24 Dec 2023]. Available from URL: https://www.has-sante.fr/jcms/p_3288393/fr/exploration- des-pathologies-thyroidiennes-chez-l-adulte-pertinence-et-criteres-de-qualite- de-l-echographie-pertinence-de-la-cytoponction-echoguidee

8. Singaporewalla RM, Hwee J, Lang TU, Desai V. Clinico-pathological correlation of thyroid nodule ultrasound and cytology using the TIRADS and

bethesda classifications. World J Surg. 2017 Jul;41(7):1807-11.
9. Russ G, Bonnema SJ, Erdogan MF, Durante C, Ngu R, Leenhardt L. European thyroid association guidelines for ultrasound malignancy risk stratification of thyroid nodules in adults: the EU-TIRADS. Eur Thyroid J. 2017 Sep;6(5):225-37.
10. Słowińska Klencka D, Wysocka Konieczna K, Klencki M, Popowicz B. Usability of EU-TIRADS in the diagnostics of hürthle cell thyroid nodules with equivocal cytology. J Clin Med. 2020 Oct;9(11):3410.
11. Kovatcheva RD, Shinkov AD, Dimitrova ID, Ivanova RB, Vidinov KN, Ivanova RS. Evaluation of the diagnostic performance of EU-TIRADS in discriminating benign from malignant thyroid nodules: a prospective study in one referral centre. Eur Thyroid J. 2021 Feb;9(6):304-12.
12. Filali SM. Intérêt du score echographique ti-rads dans la prise en charge des goitres nodulaires (à propos de 46 cas) [thesis: medicine]. Fès : Sidi Mohamed Ben Abdellah University; 2018.
13. Chatti H, Oueslati I, Marrakchi J, Azaiez A, Yazidi M, Besbes G, et al. Comparison of the diagnostic performance of ACR-TIRADS and EU-TIRADS in predicting the malignancy of thyroid nodules. Ann Endocrinol. Oct 2021;82(5):259.
14. Castellana M, Grani G, Radzina M, Guerra V, Giovanella L, Deandrea M, et al. Performance of EU-TIRADS in malignancy risk stratification of thyroid nodules: a meta-analysis. Eur J Endocrinol. 2020 Sep;183(3):255-64.
15. Hasnaoui M, Masmoudi M, Belaid T, Mighri K. Place of the TIRADS classification in the stratification of the risk of malignancy of a thyroid nodule. Ann Endocrinol. Sept 2020;81(4):228.
16. Dobruch Sobczak K, Adamczewski Z, Szczepanek Parulska E, Migda B, Woliński K, Krauze A, et al. Histopathological verification of the diagnostic performance of the EU-TIRADS classification of thyroid nodules-results of a multicenter study performed in a previously iodine-deficient region. J Clin Med. 2019 Oct;8(11):1781.

17. Myzia J, Albarel F, Paladino N, Morange I, Guerin C, Castinetti F, et al. Ultrasonographic and cytological characteristics of thyroid nodules at the Marseille University Hospital: retrospective study of 594 patients. Ann Endocrinol. Sept 2020;81(4):167.
18. Sillery JC, Reading CC, Charboneau JW, Henrichsen TL, Hay ID, Mandrekar JN. Thyroid follicular carcinoma: sonographic features of 50 cases. Am J Roentgenol. 2010 Jan;194(1):44-54.
19. Haugen BR. 2015 American thyroid association management guidelines for adult patients with thyroid nodules and differentiated thyroid cancer: what is new and what has changed: ATA 2015 thyroid nodule/DTC guidelines. Cancer. 2017 Feb;123(3):372-81.
20. Solymosi T, Hegedüs L, Bodor M, Nagy EV. EU-TIRADS-based omission of fine- needle aspiration and cytology from thyroid nodules overlooks a substantial number of follicular thyroid cancers. Int J Endocrinol. 2021 Sep;2021:1-9.
21. Zhu J, Li X, Wei X, Yang X, Zhao J, Zhang S, et al. The application value of modified thyroid imaging report and data system in diagnosing medullary thyroid carcinoma. Cancer Med. 2019 Jul;8(7):3389-400.
22. Jiang L, Zhu HB, Liang ZW, Chen L, Sun XM, Shao YH, et al. Comparison of the diagnostic performance and clinical role of different ultrasound-based thyroid malignancy risk stratification systems for medullary thyroid carcinoma. Quant Imaging Med Surg. 2023 Jun;13(6):3776-88.
23. Xu T, Wu Y, Wu RX, Zhang YZ, Gu JY, Ye XH, et al. Validation and comparison of three newly-released thyroid imaging reporting and data systems for cancer risk determination. Endocrine. 2019 May;64(2):299-307.
24. Koc AM, Adıbelli ZH, Erkul Z, Sahin Y, Dilek I. Comparison of diagnostic accuracy of ACR-TIRADS, American thyroid association (ATA), and EU-TIRADS guidelines in detecting thyroid malignancy. Eur J Radiol. 2020 Dec:133:109390.

25. Jin Z, Pei S, Shen H, Ouyang L, Zhang L, Mo X, et al. Comparative study of C- TIRADS, ACR-TIRADS, and EU-TIRADS for diagnosis and management of thyroid nodules. Acad Radiol. 2023 Oct;30(10):2181-91.
26. Hong MJ, Na DG, Baek JH, Sung JY, Kim JH. Impact of nodule size on malignancy risk differs according to the ultrasonography pattern of thyroid nodules. Korean J Radiol. 2018 May;19(3):534-41.
27. Cavallo A, Johnson DN, White MG, Siddiqui S, Antic T, Mathew M, et al. Thyroid nodule size at ultrasound as a predictor of malignancy and final pathologic size. Thyroid. 2017 May;27(5):641-50.
28. Cho MJ, Han K, Shin I, Kim EK, Moon HJ, Yoon JH, et al. Intranodular vascularity may be useful in predicting malignancy in thyroid nodules with the intermediate suspicion pattern of the 2015 American thyroid association guidelines. Ultrasound Med Biol. 2020 Jun;46(6):1373-9.
29. Kornelius E, Lo SC, Huang CN, Yang YS. The risk of thyroid cancer in patients with thyroid nodule 3 Cm or larger. Endocr Pract. 2020 Nov;26(11):1286-90.
30. Tuli G, Munarin J, Scollo M, Quaglino F, De Sanctis L. Evaluation of the efficacy of EU-TIRADS and ACR-TIRADS in risk stratification of pediatric patients with thyroid nodules. Front Endocrinol. 2022 Nov;13:1041464.
31. Hepsen S, Bostan H, Akhanli P, Sencar ME, Kizilgul M, Ucan B, et al. Subacute thyroiditis paranchime heterogeneity may mask thyroid nodules and higher EU- TIRADS scores. Endocrine. 2022 Aug;77(2):291-6.
32. Szczepanek Parulska E, Wolinski K, Dobruch Sobczak K, Antosik P, Ostalowska A, Krauze A, et al. S-detect software vs. EU-TIRADS classification: a dual-center validation of diagnostic performance in differentiation of thyroid nodules. J Clin Med. 2020 Aug;9(8):2495.
33. Cao CD, Haissaguerre M, Lussey Lepoutre C, Donatini G, Raverot V, Russ G. SFE-AFCE-SFMN 2022 consensus on the management of thyroid nodules [Online]. July 2022 [Accessed 24 Dec 2023]; [20 pages]. Available from: https://www.sfendocrino.org/wp-content/uploads/2022/08/Chapitre-2-

evaluation-initiale-Avec-filrane.pdf
34. Shi YX, Chen L, Liu YC, Zhan J, Diao XH, Fang L, et al. Differences among the thyroid imaging reporting and data system proposed by Korean, the American college of radiology and the European thyroid association in the diagnostic performance of thyroid nodules. Transl Cancer Res. 2020 Aug;9(8):4958-67.
35. Leenhardt L, Grosclaude P. Epidemiology of thyroid cancer worldwide. Ann Endocrinol. Apr 2011;72(2):136-48.
36. Tramalloni J, Monpeyssen H, Bléry M. Échographie de la thyroïde. 2ème ed. Issy- les-Moulineaux: Elsevier-Masson; 2013.
37. Clerc J. Thyroid nodule: thyroid pathology. Rev Prat. May 2005;55(2):137-48.
38. Russ G. Thyroid nodule: EU-TIRADS classification 2017 [Online]. May 2017 [Accessed the 24 Dec 2023]; [63 pages].Available at à the URL: https://www.cireol.net/wp-content/uploads/2017/05/2017-CIREOL-EUTIRADS.pdf
39. Russ G. Risk stratification of thyroid nodules on ultrasonography with the French TI-RADS: description and reflections. Ultrasonography. 2016 Jan;35(1):25-38.
40. Wémeau JL, Caron P, Schvartz C, Schlienger JL, Orgiazzi J, Cousty C, et al. Effects of thyroid-stimulating hormone suppression with levothyroxine in reducing the volume of solitary thyroid nodules and improving extranodular non-palpable changes: a randomized, double-blind, placebo-controlled trial by the french thyroid research group. J Clin Endocrinol Metab. 2002 Nov;87(11):4928-34.
41. Maino F, Forleo R, Martinelli M, Fralassi N, Barbato F, Pilli T, et al. Prospective validation of ATA and ETA sonographic pattern risk of thyroid nodules selected for FNAC. J Clin Endocrinol Metab. 2018 Jun;103(6):2362-8.
42. Tugendsam C, Petz V, Buchinger W, Schmoll Hauer B, Schenk IP, Rudolph K, et al. Ultrasound criteria for risk stratification of thyroid nodules in the

previously iodine deficient area of Austria - a single centre, retrospective analysis. Thyroid Res. 2018 May;11:3.
43. Ha SM, Kim JK, Baek JH. Detection of malignancy among suspicious thyroid nodules <1 cm on ultrasound with various thyroid image reporting and data systems. Thyroid. 2017 Oct;27(10):1307-15.
44. Peccin S, De Castro JS, Furlanetto TW, Furtado AA, Brasil BA, Czepielewski MA. Ultrasonography: is it useful in the diagnosis of cancer in thyroid nodules? J Endocrinol Invest. 2002 Jan;25(1):39-43.
45. Rayar V, Arimappamagan A, Viswanathan S, Venkatesh KD. Ultrasound and colour doppler evaluation of nodular thyroid masses. Surg Radiol Anat. 2021 Jan;10(1):17-21.
46. Peix JL, Lifante JC. Cervical curage and thyroid cancer. Ann Chir. Sept 2003;128(7):468-74.
47. Remonti LR, Kramer CK, Leitão CB, Pinto LF, Gross JL. Thyroid ultrasound features and risk of carcinoma: a systematic review and meta-analysis of observational studies. Thyroid. 2015 May;25(5):538-50.
48. Brito JP, Gionfriddo MR, Al Nofal A, Boehmer KR, Leppin AL, Reading C, et al. The accuracy of thyroid nodule ultrasound to predict thyroid cancer: systematic review and meta-analysis. J Clin Endocrinol Metab. 2014 Apr;99(4):1253-63.
49. Cappelli C, Castellano M, Pirola I, Gandossi E, De Martino E, Cumetti D, et al. Thyroid nodule shape suggests malignancy. Eur J Endocrinol. 2006 Jul;155(1):27-31.
50. Liénart F. The thyroid nodule: benign or malignant? Rev Med Brux. 2012 Sep;33(4):254-62.
51. Granja F, Morari J, Morari EC, Correa LC, Assumpção LM, Ward LS. GST profiling may be useful in the screening for thyroid nodule malignancy. Cancer Lett. 2004 Jun;209(2):129-37.

52. Frates MC, Benson CB, Charboneau JW, Cibas ES, Clark OH, Coleman BG, et al. Management of thyroid nodules detected at US: society of radiologists in ultrasound consensus conference statement. Radiology. 2005 Dec;237(3):794-800.

APPENDICES

Appendix 1-: Data collection form

Operation sheet :

1- Last name:

2- First name :

3- Geographical origin :

4- Sex: M /_/ F /_/

5- Age :

6- History:

Cervical irradiationyes /_/No /_/

Personal history of thyroid surgeryyes /_/ No /_/

Family history of thyroid neoplasia/NEMYes /_/ No /_/

Eating habitssalt /_/low-salt/_/

7- Fixed-term contract: overdraft circumstance :

Incidental /_/Anterior cervical swelling /_/ Other: specify

Time to consultation: between first symptom and consultation

8- Associated functional signs :

Signs of dysthyroidismyes /_/No /_/

If yes:hypothyroidism /_/hyperthyroidism /_/

Dysphonia :yes /_/No/_/

Dysphagia:yes /_/No /_/

Dyspnoea:yes /_/No /_/

Other: please specify

9- Physical signs :

Characteristics of the nodule :

Size :

Consistencysoft /_/firm/_/ hard/_/

Painful :yes /_/No/_/

Mobility during swallowing : mobile /_/fixed/_/

Net limits:yes /_/No /_/

Presence of cervical adenopathy:yes/_/ No/_/

If yes, which lymph nodes:

Number :

Size :

Laterality :homolateral/contralateral /Bilateral/ /

Consistency :

Mobility in relation to the two planes:mobile / /fixed //

Vocal cord mobility abnormalitiesyes /_/No /_/

If yesunilateral /_/Bilateral /_/

10- Cervical ultrasound: Thyroid volume Number

Seat left lobe / right lobe / /isthmus

Nodule size :

EchostructureAnoechoic /_/moderemebtHypoechoicIsooechoic /_/

Hyperechoic /_/very hypoechoic

Macrocalcifications:yes /_/No /_/

Microcalcifications:yes /_/No /_/

Contours :irregular /_/regular/_/

Perinodular halo:yes /_/No /_/

If yes:complete /_/incomplete /_/**Vascularisation**:central /_/

peripheral/_/mixed/_/ absent /_/

Cervical adenopathy :yes /_/No /_/

If yes, which lymph nodes:

EU_ TIRADS score classification:1 /_/2 /_/3 /_/4/_/5/_/

Thyroid BILAn :

Thyrocalcitonian

11- Fine needle aspiration: *

Not significant/_/

Benign/_/

Follicular lesion or atypia of undetermined significance/_/

Follicular neoplasm/_ /

Suspected malignancy/_/

Malignant/_ /

12- Initial surgical procedure :

Total thyroidectomy/_/loboisthmectomy/_/

Unilateral **recurrential curettage** /_/Bilateral /_/ Lateral **curageUnilateral**

Bilateral/_/

11-Exam :

Benin :/_ /

Waiting for Definitive Anapathy (ARAP):/_/Malignant:/

12-Anatomopathological examination of the surgical specimen :

Benign/_/

Malignant: Capsular rupture: yes /_/ no /_/ , **Vascular emboli**: yes /_/ no/_/ .

N0: yes /_/ no /_/ , **N+**: yes /_/ no/_/ Papillary **carcinoma/_/** Variant:

Vesicular carcinoma/_/

Medullary carcinoma/_/

Anaplastic carcinoma/_/

Others:

13-Additional surgical procedure :

Total :/_/

Contralateral recurrential curage :/_/ :

Functional curageunilateral/_/bilateral/_/ Complications of functional curage :

-Vascular :yes/ /no / /

Nerve: yes /no/ / If yes, specify the nerve affected:

Chin ramus of the facial nerve / /Spinal nerve/Phrenic//Vagus/Cervical sympathetic chain//

Lymphorrhagiayes/ no//

14-Secondary anatomopathological examination: Benign :

Clever :

Specify the histological type :

15-IRAtherapy :

Number of treatments:

Dose for each course of treatment:

16-OPPOreplacement therapy: /_/.

Appendix 2: EUTIRADS 2017 classification algorithm

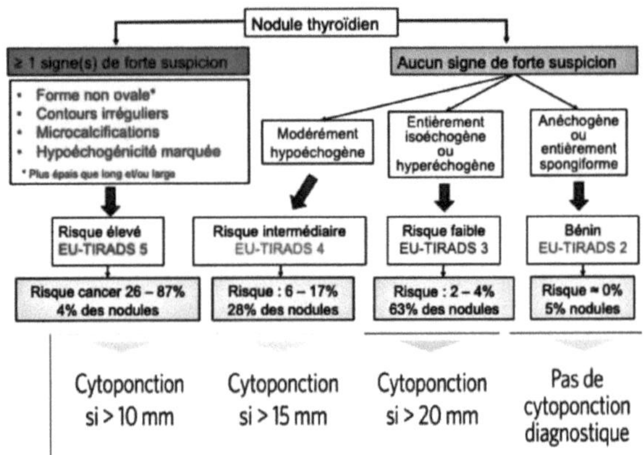

Appendix 3: Bethesda classification 2017

Bethesda 2017: risque de malignité et recommandations pour la prise en charge du patient

Catégorie diagnostique	*Risque de malignité Si NIFT-P≠ K(%)*	*Risque de malignité Si NIFT-P= K(%)*	*Prise en charge*
Non diagnostique	5-10	5-10	Deuxième ponction et US
Bénin	0-3	0-3	Suivi clinique et échographique
Atypies de signification indéterminée ou Lésion folliculaire de signification indéterminée	6-18	10-30	Deuxième ponction , test moléculaire ou lobectomie
Néoplasme folliculaire	10-40	25-40	test moléculaire ou lobectomie
Suspect de malignité	45-60	50-75	Thyroïdectomie totale ou lobectomie
Malin	94-96	97-99	Thyroïdectomie totale ou lobectomie

Appendix 4: Stratification of the risk of relapse (French society endocrinology)

		Tous les critères	Risque récurrence
Faible risque	Papillaire	• Pas d'extension extra-thyroïdienne	1-6%
		• R0	
		• N0 ou N1< 5 métastases < 2 mm	
		• M0	
		• Pas d'invasion vasculaire	
		• Pas d'histologie agressive	
		• BRAFV600E uniquement si < 1 cm	
	Vésiculaire	• Intrathyroïdien	2-3%
		• Invasion capsulaire	
		• Invasion vasculaire minime (<4 foyers)	
		1 critères parmi	**Risque récurrence**
Risque intermédiaire	Papillaire	• Invasion microscopique tissu péri thyroïdien	3-8%
		• Symptômes	9%
		• BRAFV600E uniquement si < 4cm	10%
		• Histologie agressive	15%
		• Invasion vasculaire	15-30%
		• MicroCP multifocal avec extension extra thyroïdienne BRAFV6003	20%
		• N1 clinique ou > 5 N+ (< 3cm)	20%
		• Métastase ganglionnaire fixant l'Iode	
	Vésiculaire	• N1 clinique ou > 5 N+ (< 3cm)	20%
		• Métastase ganglionnaire fixant l'Iode	
		1 critères parmi	**Risque recurrence**
Haut risque	**Papillaire**	• Extension extra-thyroïdienne macroscopique	30-40%
		• N1 > 3 cm	30%
		• Extension extra ganglionnaire	40%
		• BRAFV600E + TERT	>40%
		• Tg post op évoquant des métastases à distance	100%
		• R1	100%
		• M+	100%
	Vésiculaire	• Invasion vasculaire extensive (> 4 foyers)	30-55%
		• Tg post op évoquant des métastases à	100%
		distance	100%
		• R1	100%
		• M+	

THYROID NODULES: ECHO-HISTOLOGICAL CONFROTATION

ABSTRACT

Background :

Nodular thyroid pathology is a frequent situation in ENT practice. The EU-Tirads 2017 ultrasound classification of thyroid nodules makes it possible to predict the degree of malignancy and thus minimize unnecessary thyroid surgeries. Our aim was to study the validity of the EU-Tirads 2017 ultrasound classification by performing a histological radio comparison.

Methods :

We conducted a retrospective study involving 300 patients operated on for a nodular thyroid pathology and having previously benefited from a thyroid ultrasound using the EUTIRADS 2017 classification, all patients were treated at the ENT and CCF department of the hospital Mohamed Taher Maâmouri Nabeul during the period from 2017 to 2020.

Results :

The average age of the patients was 47.04 years. A clear female predominance was noted. Anterior basicervical swelling was the most common reason for consultation. The physical examination found a firm anterior basicervical-swelling mobile on swallowing in 94% of cases, associated with ipsilateral adenomegaly in 2.3% of cases. On cervical ultrasound, the nodules were classified EUTIRADS 2,3,4 and 5 in 0.7%, 33.3%, 39%, and 27% of cases respectively. At the end of the analytical study, we found malignancy prediction percentages of 0%, 22.1%, 41.4% and 36.4% for nodules classified EUTIRADS 2,3,4 and 5 respectively. We noted a statistically significant association of prediction of malignancy for the EUTIRADS 5 score with specificity and sensitivity equal to 36.4% and 80.3% respectively. Two criteria of score 5, namely strong hypoechogenicity and irregular contours, were significantly associated with malignancy with sensitivities of 85.2% and 62% respectively and specificities of 43.3% and 76.5% respectively. We noted that the association of at least two EUTIRADS 5 criteria was related to the higher percentage of malignancy compared to a single criterion.

Conclusion:

The Eu-Tirads 2017 ultrasound system remains extremely useful and valid for the prediction of malignancy of thyroid nodules. It helps avoid unnecessary thyroid surgeries.

Key-words: Thyroid nodule, Ultrasound, Classification, Sensitivity, Reliability and Validity, Pathological Anatomy

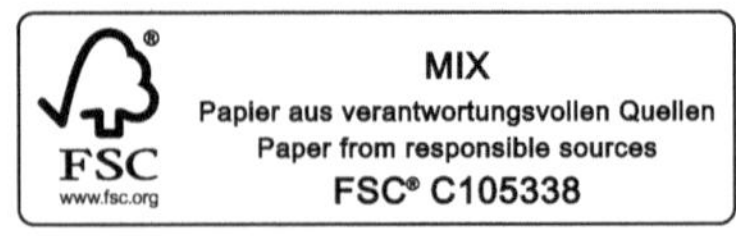

Printed by Books on Demand GmbH, Norderstedt / Germany